Fuck Fat!

How Everyday Guy's Over 50 are Losing Weight &
Changing Their Lives

Table of Contents

Brad's Story

Brad's idea of fitness is hefting the TV remote in one hand and a Big Gulp loaded with Diet Coke in the other. Up until five weeks ago he hadn't seen the inside of a gym since he was in his early thirties.

Today Brad is 55. His weight is hovering just below 400 pounds.

Brad knows the deck is stacked against him and a long life isn't in the cards for him unless he loses the excess baggage around his waist. His real problem is getting motivated to make the changes he knows he has to make.

He blames most of his problems on the hand life dealt him. He's got two teenage kids at home, a wife who's still in college, and no job. To make matters worse he doesn't have any health insurance so medical advice and prescriptions are out of the question.

Many times Brad thinks he can feel the fat piling on around his waist and chest. He often gets winded climbing up and down the steps and when he goes to the store it hurts his back, legs, and feet if he has to walk very far.

Trying to sleep at night isn't a picnic either. When he lies down in bed he has to prop his body into position with three pillows or he can't get comfortable. Even then it's hard to sleep. Most of the time he just gives up trying to fall asleep in bed and goes out and sleeps sitting up in his chair.

This has been his daily routine for at least five years now.

There are a lot of days Brad is sure he's going to die. He ends up running for the aspirin bottle hoping it can stave off the impending heart attack or stroke he feels coming on.

Five weeks ago he finally got tired of it all and decided it was time for a change.

The first thing to go was the Diet Coke.

Over the years Brad had tried to give up the soda habit with varying degrees of success. One time he actually stopped for three weeks but then habit took over and he was soon back on the bottle.

Brad decided if he could muster up the will power to give up soda it would give him the added motivation to cut back on food.

Brad had been hooked on pop since 7-Eleven came to the area in 1977. It started out as a Pepsi addiction. He spent the summer of 1979 living at home with his parents and gained 30 pounds. When he went back to school that fall he made the switch to Diet Pepsi and several years later to Diet Coke.

It's been five weeks now. He quit cold turkey and just decided to live with the headaches that giving up caffeine caused. Most of them disappeared after about two weeks.

Three weeks ago he added exercise to his routine. The first week he walked a half mile a day. It hurt his feet. Often times he found himself panting and out of breath, especially the first few days. By the end of week two he was able to walk a full mile most days. It took 39 minutes but he did it.

On week five he added light weight training.

The first thing he did was join a gym. The first two days he pulled his car into the parking lot but he was afraid to get out of his car and walk into the gym. The third day he went inside. He walked a mile, this time in 33 minutes. Then he hefted some weights. He kept them light and did ten reps.

Brad actually went into the gym three more times that week. He still hesitated in the parking lot every morning and had to talk himself into going inside each time. He constantly had the feeling people were watching him and laughing at him.

Saturday Brad weighed himself for the first time since he started making all of these changes. He weighed in at 369 pounds, down 14 pounds from the 383 pounds that he started at.

Brad has 165 pounds to go yet to reach his target weight of 205 pounds.

Read this first

Aging can make it seem like your body is launching a multi-pronged attack against you.

You know that feeling you get when you've been under siege by the flu for the last 72 hours. Aging can literally take you through the wringer just like that and leave you feeling drained and lifeless.

Here is what's really happening ...

As you age your heart rate gradually begins to slow down and your heart may even start to get bigger. As this happens your blood vessels can start to harden. This is what can eventually lead to hypertension (high blood pressure).

Another problem men face as they age is their bones can actually begin to shrink, not just in size, but also in density. This can lead to osteoporosis and weaker bones that can fracture more easily.

At the same time your muscles are beginning to get weaker and less flexible so it becomes more painful to stretch and move around.

Aging can also put extra stress on *The Little General* making it harder for him to perform. Erections can take longer to achieve or may not last as long. Ejaculations can become smaller, decreasing sexual pleasure.

To top it off aging can play tricks with your mental acuity. As a result, brain farts, those unpleasant moments where you spaz out or have to think things out for an extra second or two can become more common.

You have the Power to Turn Back Aging …

Many people deny it. They say "it's bound to happen," but the truth is Smoky the Bear had it right, "only you can prevent the horrors of aging or turn the clock back on it."

Medical study after medical study has shown that by eating right and getting moderate exercise you can reset your internal clock by 20 years or more.

What this means is that with a little TLC you can be healthier at fifty than you were at thirty.

If it's so easy, what's holding people back?

That's a good question. Most people live their life in fear of change. Let's go back to Brad in our first example.

Brad watched himself pack on the weight. He knew it was causing him untold problems, not to mention all of the hours of lost sleep. No matter what happened he kept telling himself – "Just one more bucket of chicken." "I'll eat this last bag of candy, and then I can start my diet."

Sounds familiar, doesn't it?

Each time he tried to break off his love affair with Diet Coke he told himself, "just one more, and then I'm done."

For three years in a row his New Year's Resolution was to give up soda. Every year when the time came he told himself he'd have just one more on the First because it was a holiday, and then he was done.

Of course you know how that turned out. He decided he'd just drink pop the first week, then the first month, then...

Life happens, and we tell ourselves stories

One of them is, "I will get started on that tomorrow," but tomorrow never comes.

Jim's Story

Jim was always a little over weight.

"I was six foot tall and two hundred pounds when I started the sixth grade," he jokes. "I just sort of grew up, and grew out that summer.

"When I got to junior high and high school all of the coaches wanted me to wrestle or play football but sports weren't my thing.

"I liked to sit at home and read books. I think stamp collecting was my favorite thing then. I was sure I was going to be a stamp dealer. I read everything about stamp collecting – books, price guides, magazines.

"I didn't have many friends. Most of the guys made fun of me because of my size so I stayed to myself.

"I went off to college in 1976. It was a big school with a campus that spread out over several miles so I had to do a lot of walking to get from class to class. When we went out at night no one had a car so we had to walk downtown to the bars.

"Anyway when I went back to my parent's house the following summer everyone started commenting on how much I'd changed and how much thinner I looked.

After I heard it enough I decided to step on a scale and see for myself what they were talking about. I weighed 195 pounds; when I left for school the year before I was 247 pounds.

"I never noticed I'd changed or lost weight. Even when I looked in the mirror I still saw that same old fat kid the guys made fun of back in high school."

Jim kept the weight off through all of his time in school and for most of the next decade.

He got married when he was thirty-two; had his first kid when he was thirty-five; and another when he was thirty-seven. When he was thirty-eight his work made some changes and he was transferred from the Midwest to the west coast. The first five weeks he flew back and forth every week so he was always eating out or on the run.

When they moved they spent their first three months living out of motel rooms waiting for the house to be finished. That meant more restaurant food for every meal and constant snacks in between.

After they moved into their new house this pattern just sort of continued on. Rather than eat at home they found it more convenient to eat out. It was riblets at Applebee's; enchiladas at Chi-Chi's; Chinese at the Panda Express; but their favorite place to eat was at buffets.

For the next fifteen years they feasted at buffets a minimum of two days a week.

Over the next fifteen years Jim and his wife doubled in size. He was now fifty-three and 350 pounds. She was forty-eight and 257 pounds.

Like most people Jim and his wife saw it happening. They just couldn't stop themselves. Going out to eat and hitting the buffets had become a regular part of their lives.

Although they didn't know it yet that behavior was slowly killing them and their children.

The first indication Jim had that he was really in trouble happened two years ago when he was sitting at his computer.

*"All of a sudden I felt two electrical shocks just above my heart," Jim explained it. "I was just sitting there typing away - no pain or problems, and **wham – wham**. Several minutes later it happened again, and then again.*

"I wasn't short of breath. I wasn't sweating, but I was having chest pains. I grabbed a bottle of aspirins and swallowed a few just in case. Then I had my wife take me to emergency. They kept me there overnight.

"It wasn't a heart attack but I kept having chest pains. They did a stress test and an echocardiogram. There was no heart damage but the chest pains persisted.

"When it was all said and done the doctors decided I probably had GERD and gave me some medicine for that. They also discovered my blood pressure was out there in the stratosphere. It was 181 over 110. I was a heart attack or stroke waiting to happen.

"They made it clear this was my wake-up-call. I needed to lose weight if I wanted to live to see sixty."

After that Jim started making some simple changes to his lifestyle. He went on a diet.

Being on a diet was hard for Jim.

Giving up restaurants was just as hard. A lot of times he fell off of the wagon, especially when his wife and kids are snacks or goodies in front of him. Life seemed unfair.

Jim kept at it. If he fell down for a day or two and ate the wrong foods he would always pick himself up and get started again.

He started walking the dog. At first they took short walks. As Jim and the dog adjusted to it they walked farther and farther. Within a month they were walking two miles a day.

After two months Jim and the dog were walking before he went to work in the morning and again when he came home from work at night. Most days they logged five miles.

At the end of month three Jim had to buy new clothes for the second time since he started walking. He'd lost 29 pounds, but the most exciting thing for him was dropping four pants sizes. He went from a 48 to 44 waist size.

The next thing Jim did was talk to his doctor about lifting weights. The doctor thought it was a good idea but urged him to start out slow and not to push it.

Jim bought some dumbbells and worked out with them three days a week. He definitely wasn't any Arnold Schwarzenegger, but after a few months he did feel stronger.

Another thing Jim noticed was he wasn't huffing and puffing on the stairs anymore or out of breath after crossing a parking lot.

"I gave myself cheat days," said Jim. "I decided one day a week, I could eat fried chicken or hit the buffet. That way it didn't feel like I was giving up all of the foods I liked."

Today Jim is fifty-five years old. He weighs 215 pounds and he's in the best shape he's been in since his college years.

His last piece of advice is, "Always pick yourself up after the fall. Everyone's going to overeat one day or skip a workout. Don't worry about it! Just get started again the next day."

Step # 1 - You need to change the way you think

Like Jim you're going to discover the hardest part of getting fit is changing the way you think.

Over the years you build up a set of habits...

You get up in the morning and get ready for work. You hop in the car and head off to the Kwik Shop for a Soda and a donut or breakfast sandwich. Somewhere around midmorning you make a pit stop at the bathroom and the vending machines are begging you to get a candy bar.

What's a guy going to do? You buy a candy bar.

By noon it's time for lunch. You get in your car and head for McDonald's or Arby's, and then it's back to work.

On the way home you pull into the Kwik Shop for a giant sized soda and a snack to carry you through the evening.

You could even argue it's not your fault that you do these things. The car has a habit of stopping there. You're just along for the ride.

I understand.

We're all creatures of habit!

It's part of being human. If you do something enough it becomes a routine part of your life.

I have a dog. He's an American Eskimo. Whenever anyone is in the kitchen making food he makes his way over to the scene of the action waiting for fall out and handouts.

Over the years he's learned he's going to get a few samples and when he's really lucky some crumbs will make their way to the floor. He just needs to be there waiting for them.

When the action switches to the dining room table he makes his way over there, and waits and waits, because he knows someone's going to share their food with him.

People are no different than their pets...

The dog knows if he hangs out where the food is, he's bound to get some. So what does he do, he makes sure he's in the best position to get his share.

As people we do the same thing.

We put ourselves in the position where we're most likely to eat, even when we're trying to stop.

I've got this thing for those mini cherry pies they sell at Wal-Mart. I know I shouldn't but every time I go to Wal-Mart I pick up three or four of those mini cherry pies. I tell myself I'm just going to have one of them every day for breakfast.

Can anybody guess what happens?

Not hard to figure, is it? I eat at least two of them.

So what's a guy to do?

We're often our own worst enemies. We set ourselves up to fail. As humans, it's what we do.

I'm going to share this secret with you...

The *free dictionary* defines willpower as: *The strength of will to carry out one's decisions, wishes, or plans.*

Losing weight takes will power. Lots of willpower or it's not going to happen.

All of us have the will power to do whatever we want.

Some people get inspired. For others the will power comes to them when the doctor says "lose weight, or die."

I had the will power twenty-five years ago and lost 108 pounds in thirteen months. I told myself I was through with the madness. I wrote down every ounce of food I put in my mouth. I started working out every day and the weight just fell off.

You need to make it fun!

Sometimes we need a little help.

I used to work at a car dealership. One of the managers there wanted to lose weight but he knew he needed a little help staying motivated so he came up with a contest.

He got twelve of us to kick in $20.00 each. Every week, for eight weeks we got together on Monday mornings for a weigh in. Anyone who gained weight had to toss in $10.00.

Along the way half of the people dropped out but for the ones who kept the game in play it was a great motivator not to mention a money maker. By the time the contest ended there was over $500.00 in the kitty.

If all else fails, bribe yourself...

When we were potty training my oldest daughter it seemed like she would never get the hang of it. Then my wife had this light bulb idea. We bought a couple boxes of Pokémon cards on eBay.

Every time she used the big people's potty my daughter got a pack of Pokémon cards. It was just the motivator she needed and we could finally stop buying all of those diapers.

When it was my second daughter's time to potty train we knew exactly what to do.

What's your price?

Have you always wanted to pick out a new wardrobe? Perhaps you have your eye on an iPad? Or even a new car?

Ask yourself what it's going to take to keep you motivated and make yourself a promise that you're going to do it.

PS: A car is a great motivator but if you promise yourself a major prize (like a car or a whirlwind trip around the world) at the end of the journey you need to make sure it is doable. The last thing you want to do is promise yourself something that is impossible to deliver on or unaffordable. If you do this you will find yourself quitting at the first speed bump you encounter.

Create plenty of smaller milestones...

Don't just dangle a big carrot out there at the end of the road. Treat yourself to plenty of smaller rewards along the way. It will help keep you pumped up and motivated along the way.

Let's say you're like Brad and you have 179 pounds to lose. A shiny new BMW would certainly motivate anyone, but Brad's journey is going to be a long one. He's looking at a minimum of two years, maybe more. If he's going to succeed he needs to have plenty of smaller celebrations along the way.

Think of it like sending your kid off to college. She's got four years of school ahead of her. The carrot the school dangles in front of her is always the degree, but they're careful to offer plenty of feedback along the way. Over the four years your daughter is attending that college she will complete eight semesters of classes. Each semester she will receive feedback (grades) that let her know how she is doing. By monitoring her feedback she can adjust her study habits to ensure she succeeds.

You need to set your fitness program up the same way.

Celebrate the first five pounds you lose. Celebrate every twenty-five pounds along the way. Or if you want to celebrate differently, get excited every time that you drop a clothes size. Jim, in our second example, went from a size 48 waist to a size 34 waist. His shirt size dropped from a 5 XL to a XL. When it was all said and done, Jim didn't have to shop for clothes online anymore. He could find clothes that fit him at any store.

Decide what's important to you and set smaller milestones that are reachable. Don't make them too easy; at the same time don't make them unachievable.

Too many people set themselves up to fail. Make sure you set yourself up to succeed.

Barry's Story

Barry has been active all of his life. He's fifty-two. In the summer he plays golf at least five days a week.

"Not that wimpy game where they ride along in the cart and just get out to tap the ball around," says Barry. "I walk the course, up and down the hills, and along the trails back to the club house.

"I'm not one of those guys who start out with a beer in the club house, stash a twelve-pack in the golf cart, and meet up at the nineteenth hole after the game to swap stories over even more beer.

"That's not golf! That's a bunch of guys making excuses to drink."

Barry is in pretty good shape overall. At six foot, three inches tall, he weighs 245 pounds. His problem is his belly. It just seems to keep getting a little bigger.

Three months ago his doctor told Barry he had high blood pressure and his HDL cholesterol was a little low. The doctor put him on Toprol and Benicar for his blood pressure and Crestor to help control his cholesterol.

Barry had never had to take regular prescriptions before except for antibiotics now and then to combat frequent bouts of sinusitis. The thought of taking medicines for the rest of his life bothered Barry.

He did a lot of research on the internet. One of the things he discovered was it was possible to regulate his blood pressure through proper diet and exercise. Barry talked with his doctor again, and he agreed diet and exercise could work for Barry if he stuck with it. One of the smartest things his doctor did was have him talk to a nutritionist. Together they put together an eating plan to help him achieve his goals.

That visit to the nutritionist was a real eye opener for Barry. She told him a normal portion of meat was about the size of a deck of cards.

The nutritionist explained to him a normal portion of steak or cooked beef was three ounces. When Barry went out to eat with his wife at the Lone Star he always had the 14 oz. Peppercorn Rib Eye. She also told him a proper portion for potatoes was one potato (about the size of a computer mouse). He was used to getting an appetizer of steak fries smothered in bacon and cheese, along with another side order of steak fries with his steak. After hearing this he didn't have the guts to ask what she thought about the Big Brownie Blast they always had for desert.

When he left the nutritionist that day Barry had the feeling he'd been doing it wrong for his entire life. Barry learned his whole philosophy of eating from TV commercials when he was growing up. Remember that Lays Potato Chip ad — "No one can eat just one!"

Barry had taken that commercial to heart. He never ate just one, even when he was full, or the food tasted just so-so.

When he got home that day Barry explained it all to his wife. He showed her the menus the nutritionist made up for him. Like Barry she had trouble grasping the idea that a normal portion was so small. Their kids had eaten more than that when they were seven or eight years old.

They talked it over that night and again the next morning. After a lot of thought they decided they would give the nutritionist's plan a try. They went grocery shopping that afternoon.

The first few weeks Barry and his wife were up and down on their diets. The hardest thing for them was going out to eat or having dinner with friends.

After about a month they began to see some progress. Barry could tighten his belt buckle another notch without having to suck in his belly, and his wife noticed her clothes fit a little looser.

Barry lost 25 pounds his first four months of dieting. More importantly when he saw his doctor they decided he could stop taking his blood pressure medicines.

The deal was he had to get a wrist monitor and check his blood pressure two or three times per week. If it started inching up he was supposed to tell the doctor.

Step 2 – It's all in how you look at it

In most cases it's not the food we eat that's unhealthy. It's how much of it we eat.

We live an age where everything we eat is supersized. You go to the 7-Eleven and you can get a Super Big Gulp (64 oz.), or even a Double Super Big Gulp (128 oz.).

According to recent studies restaurant portion sizes have doubled and even tripled over the past twenty years.

What immediately comes to mind for me is eating out at the Cheese Cake Factory. All of their portions are ginormous. When we lived in Baltimore I took all of my employees out to eat at the Cheese Cake Factory in the Harbor. There were eleven of us and every one of us ordered their own appetizer. I will never forget when they brought them out. Those appetizers filled the entire table. Two of them would have fed all of us.

That's nothing compared to when they served our deserts. I had an ice cream brownie covered in whipped cream that was big enough to feed a family of four for two days.

The enormous portions served by many restaurants have caused many of us to develop distorted views about portion sizes. Kids who've grown up over the last thirty years have become accustomed to these oversized portions and to being asked "would you like to super-size that?"

To lose weight, you need to eat less

Sounds easy, doesn't' it?

What makes losing weight hard for many of us is that we don't realize that we are over eating.

Consider the typical hamburger.

Fast food hamburgers come in many varieties - regular, quarter-pounder, third-pounder, and even half-pounder. Sometimes they call them double burgers, or triple burgers, and slip extra cheese in between each layer.

The proper portion size for a hamburger is three ounces. If you want to lose weight, and stay healthy, skip the quarter pounder. Say no way to the six dollar burger. If you must eat fast food order the regular burger off of the dollar menu. You'll save a few bucks and several hundred calories.

Here are the proper portion sizes for each of the major food groups.

Meats / Nuts

Cooked Beef - 3 oz.
Chicken Breast - 3oz.
Fish - 3 oz.
Lunch meats - 1 oz.
Nut - ¼ cup

Fruit

Apple - 1
Banana - 1
Strawberries – 1 cup
Blueberries – ½ cup
Grapes – ½ cup

Vegetables

Baked Potato - 1
Mashed potatoes – ½ cup
Corn on the cob – 1 ear
Beans / carrots / veggies – 1 cup

Grains

Bagel – 1
Bread – 1 slice
Cereal – 1 cup
Pasta – 1 cup
Popcorn – 1 cup
Rice – ½ cup

Dairy

Milk – 8 oz. cup low fat milk
Yogurt – 8 oz. cup
Cheese – 2 oz.

Sweets

Brownie – 2" square
Cake – 1" slice
Chocolate – 1 oz.
Cookie – 1 (3" round)

Ice cream – ½ cup
Pudding – 1 cup

It's sort of scary the first time you look at it.

At restaurants when they bring us chicken tenders, they normally serve five or six, not one. When they serve the brownie for desert, it's often times eight inches or larger and covered in ice cream, topped with whipped cream. When Subway makes a Foot-Longer there's definitely more than 1 ounce of lunch meat there.

It's going to take you time to adjust...

Now that you know what the proper portion size is, it's going to take some time to adjust to it.

My suggestion is to ease into it. Slowly cutting back on portion sizes over one or two weeks will give you time to adjust and make a game plan for eating healthier.

One website I would suggest visiting is Fighting Flab. The Mayo Clinic guide to portion size might help. http://www.cbsnews.com/pictures/fighting-flab-mayo-clinic-guide-to-portion-size-might-help/

It is hosted by CBS News. The nice thing they do is show you what a portion looks like. For example, a 2 oz. serving of cheese is equivalent to four pieces of cheese the same size as four dice. A serving of almonds (45 calories) is just seven almonds, and a portion of fruit such as an apple or an orange is about the size of a tennis ball or baseball.

Keep this in mind as you begin to plan a meal or look for a snack.

WebMD has designed a slick PDF you can print out to keep on your refrigerator or counter top for a quick reference. It shows you how to design your plate and gives your portion sizes, along with weights and pictures so that you can better understand them.

Bill's Story

Bill was a road warrior.

He traveled seven states oftentimes logging over 2500 miles per week. One day he'd be in Chicago, the next day he'd wake up in Des Moines, and the day after could be anybody's guess – Indianapolis, Peoria, maybe even St. Louis.

Bill lived out of his car. Whenever his cell phone rang he was off chasing his next sale.

His wakeup call happened in Milwaukee just over nine months ago. It started with some minor indigestion when he crawled out of bed that morning. He ate a couple Tums after breakfast and hit the highway heading towards Chicago. The pains nagged him all of the way there. At lunch the pains got worse; Bill started sweating, and feeling short of breath.

He doesn't remember too much else until he woke up in the hospital later that afternoon. The doctors told him they were going to do an angiogram and based on what they found they may be putting in a stent or if they found major damage they might have to do heart bypass surgery.

Bill got a few minutes to call his wife and then hoped for the best. He was lucky and got by with a stent, but the situation made Bill take a closer look at his life and what he was doing with it.

He made good money but he was always on the go. Bill never had time for himself or his family. He always had to be somewhere and he never knew where until the next phone call came in.

To sum it all up: Bill was 51 years old. He was five foot nine inches tall and weighed 275 pounds. His diet was a combination of fast food, candy bars, chips, and afternoon drinks while schmoozing with clients. In a good week he was home a day and a half and part of that time was spent on the phone and laptop confirming and expediting orders.

After his incident Bill took a few weeks off to recuperate and decide what was important to him.

With the help and encouragement of his wife Bill decided twenty-seven years on the road was long enough. It was time to slow down and change his life. Bill was lucky. His wife had a good job, they had some money in the bank, and his kids were both out of college. If he was going to make any kind of changes now was the perfect time.

Bill left his job that week and decided to give himself five or six months to reinvent his career.

One of the first things he did was to start walking. He set a goal of a mile a day his first week. After adjusting to that he bumped it up to two miles and then three. His daughter got him an Alaskan Husky to keep him company on his walks and together Bill and the dog were logging five and six miles per day by the end of his second month.

Food was another problem for Bill. Because he had spent so much time on the road he never really had time for meals. Everything he ate was something he could munch on in the car while he was driving. Making the transition to real meals gave Bill some tough choices.

During the day Bill was home alone while his wife worked. If he was still on the road he would have hit McDonalds for a burger or Arby's for chicken tenders, but now that he was home he had to fend for himself. That meant making his own meals and making smart choices about what he should eat.

That wasn't always easy for Bill. Sometimes he gave in and got fast food but most of the time he had salad or a sandwich. One of the things that helped him through were meal replacement drinks (Slim-fast and Equate) and protein bars.

Over a nine month period Bill lost 65 pounds and eight inches around his waist. Bill has 50 pounds more to go to reach his goal of 165 pounds. He figures he will reach his goal in another six to nine months.

Step 3 – The Basics

There's no magic secret for weight loss. If you are overweight, you either need to eat less, exercise more, or do a combination of these.

If you want to lose one pound you need to cut out 3500 calories.

If you want to lose ten pounds, you need to eliminate 35,000 calories (10 x 3500). Doctors say you can safely lose one to two pounds per week. Two pounds per week would require you to cut 1000 calories per day (7000 / 7). To do this you could add enough exercise to burn off 1000 calories, cut 1000 calories in food, or do a combination of each.

That's really all there is to it. If you want to lose weight, eat less, and exercise more.

So how do you get started?

Forget the latest fads. They will only work as long as you can stick to them. How long can you eat just protein, or grapefruit, or...? Fads are a temporary fix. It's going to be next to impossible to stick with a diet that won't let you eat your favorite foods.

Break it down into simple steps

1) **Visit with your doctor**. Before you begin any diet or exercise program it's important to consult with your doctor and make sure you don't have any physical conditions that will prevent you from beginning an exercise program.

2) **Consult a nutritionist**. While talking to a nutritionist isn't necessary it will give you with an entirely new outlook on the foods you eat. We've already talked about portion sizes earlier in this book. Everywhere you go they're out of control. Just about every food you buy is available in supersize, and super – supersize. A good nutritionist can help you sort it all out and plan an eating program that will give you a better shot at succeeding.

3) **Start walking**. Walking is one of the easiest exercise programs to get started with. You can walk anywhere. It's free. It doesn't require any special equipment, membership fees, or reservations. You just

need to head out the door and get started. It gets your entire body moving, and pumps up your cardiovascular system.

4) **Buy a scale**. Whether you need to lose ten pounds or one hundred pounds you need a scale to keep track of your progress. You're going to have slow weeks and slow months where no matter what you do the scale just barely budges. When that happens you can put it in perspective by looking at where you are now and where you started from.

5) **Take measurements**. Get a fabric tape measure and take measurements. Be sure to get around your waist, around your chest, your arms, your thighs, and anywhere else you want to keep track of. Some weeks, and even some months, the scale is barely going to budge. That's when the tape will take over to help you stay motivated. Keep walking and eating less and the inches will keep falling off. Take your measurements at least once a month to celebrate all of those inches you're losing.

6) **Start journaling**. Write down everything you eat. Keep a record of how far you walk or how much weight you can lift. If you're really worn out after your workout, write that down. If you feel good after your workout write that down. If you decided to try a different eating strategy record it in your journal. The more you write the more

information you will have to look over so that you can really determine what is working for you.

7) **Lift weights**. You don't have to be an Olympic weight lifter or even attempt to lift hundreds of pounds. Lifting even light amounts of weight can help firm and tone your muscles. You can join a gym or if you prefer buy some dumbbells and set up workout station in your home.

Whatever, you chose to do remember, to keep it healthy. Your goal should be regular moderate exercise.

According to the American College of Sports Medicine (ACSM) men over fifty should get from 20 to 60 minutes of cardio exercise three to five days per week. They should also workout two to three times per week.

Tom's Story

Tom was always good in sports. In high school he played on the baseball and football teams. He went on to play college football. He had hoped to go pro but a debilitating knee injury in his senior year put ended that dream.

After school he joined a large engineering company. Tom's job kept him on the move. Over the next thirty years he lived in seven different cities and visited five different countries helping to supervise projects in each of them.

No matter how busy he was Tom always made time for his workouts. When he was on the road he made sure the company booked him in hotels with a gym. Whenever he moved he made sure that the apartment buildings he lived in had their own workout centers.

Tom was an avid jogger. He often logged five miles a day or more. When the weather was bad he ran on the treadmill. He was obsessed with lifting weights. He worked out five days a week, training different segments of his body each day. Tom squatted 350 pounds and benched over 250 pounds.

Despite all of the time he spent working out Tom couldn't prevent the bulge in his abdomen from growing.

Tom kept his washboard abs into his mid-forties but as he approached fifty he noticed several changes in his appearance and in his ability to workout.

One of the things Tom noticed was he couldn't recover as quickly between workouts. The number of reps he could do was slowly creeping down, and the amount of weight he could lift was stalled out. Tom tried several different workouts but they didn't seem to help. He considered trying some supplements but decided against taking them because he'd always been a natural bodybuilder.

When none of this worked for him Tom approached a personal trainer and shared his story with him.

One of the things the trainer told Tom was that most of the problems he was experiencing were the natural results of aging. Once men turn forty it muscle mass can decline by as much as ten percent per decade. For Tom the muscle loss wasn't as devastating because he had continued to work out and keep his muscles active.

The trainer suggested Tom should tweak his exercise routine a little. "The thing is," the trainer told him, "your body will adapt to just about any routine that you throw at it. The trick is to constantly shake it up. Don't use all heavy weights. Throw in some light training days too."

Another thing the trainer reminded Tom about was that he wasn't thirty anymore. As you get older your muscles and joints aren't as limber as they used to be. Don't rush into your workout – take fifteen or twenty minutes to warm up first. That would help him prevent damaging his muscles while helping him to lift heavier weights.

The trainer also suggested Tom should limit his workouts to one hour at a time. His goal should be to get a good workout without overstressing his body. He told Tom to spend more time isolating muscle groups in his workouts.

As far as the extra bulge around his waist the trainer gave him two choices – eat less and eat smarter, or do more cardio. He agreed with Tom about not taking supplements. He told him he could get the same effects by eating properly and varying his workout.

None of this was new to Tom. He was just too busy with other things and in the resulting confusion he lost track of the basics.

Over the next three months he went back to basics. He varied his workout, isolated muscle groups, and made changes in his diet. By the start of his second month of doing this Tom began to see some changes he liked. He didn't get his washboard abs back but he was confident he could get there with a little more work.

Step 4 – How much exercise should you do?

It's never too late to start getting the benefits of exercise. Studies have shown that everyone, no matter what their age, can benefit from some form of exercise.

The benefits are not all physical. In addition to looking better and being able to move easier exercise will also:

. Increase your brain power, and prevent the onset of Alzheimer's and dementia
. Delay arterial aging (hardening and clogging of your arteries)
. Increase flexibility in your joints, for easier movement
. Increase bone strength, thus reducing your chances for suffering from osteoporosis and arthritis

Staying fit is the best way to ensure you have a better quality of life as you age.

It will enable you to continue doing the things you like such as spending more time with your children and grandchildren. It will give you more freedom in your retirement years.

To ensure you get these benefits you need to add weight lifting and cardiovascular exercises into your daily routine.

As men age weight training becomes more important. Increasing your muscular strength and flexibility doesn't mean you need to lift massive amounts of weight. It's ok to start out with lower weights doing fifteen to twenty reps, but for maximum benefits you have to test your muscles. You need to find a weight that challenges your muscles. Aim to do six to eight reps at your maxim weight.

The same goes for cardiovascular exercises. You need to find an activity you enjoy and do twenty to sixty minutes of it three to five times a week.

No matter how busy your life is it's easy to add cardio.

Here are a few things you can try:

- Take a walk at lunch time
- Take the stairs instead of the elevator
- Play softball
- Ride a bike or an exercise bike
- Park at the far end of the parking lot
- Garden
- Get up out of the chair to change the channel

Mike's story

Mike grew up in a family obsessed with food.

His parents owned a family style restaurant and once they turned ten the kids were expected to help out. He can remember most summers, he bussed tables sneaking food samples every time he passed through the kitchen.

Most days his family ate supper at the restaurant as soon as the dinner rush ended. On weekends they ate breakfast, lunch, and supper there sneaking time in between rushes. It was a crazy life and just about everything in his family's life centered round food.

The food salesmen were always bringing samples of new deserts, breads, and appetizers that they all cooked up and tried. There were deserts everywhere he looked and Mike sampled all of them.

By the time he was eighteen and getting ready to head off to college Mike weighed 325 pounds at six foot tall. His sister, Marsha, weighed 250 pounds, and his brothers were both pushing 300 pounds.

College was the first time Mike was out on his own. It was the first time he was actually away from food where it wasn't surrounding him and tempting him.

Without the constant temptations he was eating less. Mike didn't realize it yet but he was starting to lose weight. His first real clue came about a month after school started. His jeans fit better. He didn't have to suck his gut in to squeeze into them anymore. He didn't have to play all of the games he was used to when he got dressed.

Another thing he noticed was his belt was looser. In the past he'd always fought with it, trying to get in latched in the last notch. Now he could let it out one notch. He noticed the same thing with his shirts, that 5 XL was now a little baggy on him.

Without even really trying to lose weight Mike lost nearly 75 pounds his first year at college.

When he returned home that summer Mike started working at the restaurant again. It opened up a whole new can of worms for him. Everywhere he went he was surrounded by food. He wanted to eat but he also liked the new thinner Mike. Each time he caught himself grabbing for a handful of fries, or an onion ring, or a piece of pie, he had to tell himself – NO!

By the end of that summer he gained ten pounds back.

When he returned to school he started losing weight again and eventually got down to 195 pounds. After graduation he got a job in Chicago managing a retail store. It was a big box superstore and he got a lot of activity moving around it so it helped him keep in shape.

By the time he was thirty Mike got married. About that same time he decided retail management wasn't his thing. He was tired of working around people all of the time and spending all of his holidays and weekends at work.

He scored a marketing job with a large food broker. At first he spent most of his time in the office but as time went on they had him on the road most of the time doing food shows and presenting new products at restaurants with the salesmen.

It wasn't long before Mike fell back into the old routine he'd learned in his parent's restaurant. Everywhere he went he was surrounded by food. At food shows he was cooking up food and dishing out samples while he talked with customers. When he had some spare moments he was checked out the competition and sampled their newest products. After the food show ended they were checked out the new restaurants in whatever town they were in.

When he visited restaurants with his salesmen Mike was always bringing in new products to show them. One of his jobs was helping restaurant owners prepare the samples he brought to them. Mike always made plenty of food so the entire restaurant staff could sample it and of course Mike had his share as well.

It wasn't long before he started packing on the weight again. Mike knew it was happening. He told himself he needed to slow down on the food but one thing led to another. He told himself he'd get started on it tomorrow or the next day.

Unfortunately tomorrow never came. At age 51 Mike found himself pushing the scale at 355 pounds.

About that same time Mike's company encountered a few speed bumps in their growth. They were bought out by another company and the new owners phased out a lot of their private brands. They brought in more of their own people and pushed a lot of the old people out.

Mike's job was eliminated and he was out on the street.

"One of the first things I did," Mike said, "was to take a good look at my life. The last twenty years of selling on the road was the most fun I ever had. It wasn't anything like work at all. I travelled all over the country, stayed in great hotels and all I did was talk to people.

"All around me I saw all of these people working their asses off. Mom and dad, and my brothers and sisters, they worked ten, twelve hours a day, six days a week in that restaurant, and for what? A couple bucks in tips? Then they had to do it all over again the next day.

"I also looked at myself. I'd become that fat loser I was in high school. All I did anymore was talk and eat. I'm surprised my wife didn't run out the door on me years before. I was never home and when I was all I did was talk on the phone and eat.

"I decided I needed to take back my life. I bought a few books on fitness and dieting. I wasn't even smart enough to go to the doctor first. I think I was afraid he was going to tell me I was fat.

"The first thing I did was get a treadmill. After five minutes I was tired and I had to stop. Things went on like this for a week, and I think I was finally walking for maybe fifteen minutes. It made my feet sore and my head was dizzy when I got off of it.

"The second week I got a little farther. I think I was up to twenty minutes twice a day.

"Three weeks into this fitness kick I was on I started cutting back on food. At first I just cut out lunch and had a meal replacement drink instead. A few days later I started to change my snacks. Instead of a candy bar or a donut I started eating protein bars and an occasional apple or orange.

"The first month I lost twelve pounds and dropped a full pants size. I was now a 48 waist.

"That really encouraged me. I upped my walking to a half hour twice a day. At my new walking speed that was almost two and a half miles per day.

"I changed the way I was eating. When I was doing some research online I discovered this thing they call the DASH Diet. What I liked about it was it wasn't really a diet at all – in the traditional sense. It told me how many servings of what types of food I should eat. It didn't tell me to eat spinach and carrots, kumquats and liver. I could still eat the foods I liked. I just had to fit them into the food groups I was supposed to eat and stick to the proper number of servings and portion sizes. It made it easier for me.

"I kept this pace up for about six months. At the end of that time I began to see some real changes. My pants size was down to a 42 waist, and I weighed 293 pounds. I'd lost 62 pounds.

"After that I bought some weights and started working out with them in the basement. I didn't go crazy with them. I think I used them twenty or thirty minutes three days a week.

"I was feeling pretty good by this time. My feet didn't hurt when I walked anymore and I found myself doing a lot of the things I hadn't done in years. I was bending over to pick things up instead of walking by them. I even washed my car inside, and outside, all by myself.

"It's been almost a year now. I have a 38 waist size, and I weigh 248 pounds.

"If I can do it anybody can."

Step 5 – Diet is a four letter word

For most of us diet is a four letter word. It's scary and it makes us think we're going to have to torture ourselves to make it work.

One of the things the word "diet" makes me think about is I'm going to have to give up all of my favorite foods.

Every year at New Year's I tell my wife I'm going to do it. This year I'm going to give up soda and start eating right. In past years she's always just looked at me and smiled knowingly. She knew I was full of it and I wasn't really going to give up anything.

This year when I said it she took a new tact and asked, "Why don't you just decide to do something healthy instead like drink a glass of milk every day. It's healthy and it will give you more protein."

It seemed doable. I like milk and it would be pretty easy to drink a glass of it every day.

Diet doesn't mean you have to give up your favorite foods...

I think the reason so many people are afraid to go on a diet is they think they have to give up all of their favorite foods.

What I'm suggesting is you look at it a different way? What if you keep eating your favorite foods but just not as often or as much? Would that make dieting easier?

Going back to Mike's example he liked the DASH Diet because he could still eat the foods he liked. By not having to give up his favorite foods it made it easier for him to adjust to the changes he had in front of him.

One of the diets most recommended by doctors is the DASH Diet. It was originally developed to help lower blood pressure but one of the side effects researchers discovered was that when followed properly it also helps to melt off pounds

The DASH Diet is heavy on fruits and vegetables, but it gives users leeway to eat many of the foods they like as long as they eat the proper portion sizes.

A typical day on the DASH Diet looks something like this:

- Grains 6 – 12 servings
- Fruits 4 – 6 servings
- Vegetable 4 – 6 servings
- Lean or non-fat dairy products 2 – 4 servings
- Lean meats, fish, and poultry 2 – 3 servings
- Nuts, seed, legumes 1 serving
- Fats and sweets 2 – 4 servings

Your actual servings would depend upon how much weight you want to lose and how many calories you are consuming daily.

Dr. Oz gives a quick explanation of the DASH Diet here, Dr. Oz explaining the Dash Diet.

http://www.doctoroz.com/slideshow/understand-dash-diet-5-clicks?

Follow the next link to search on Amazon for good books explaining how to implement the DASH Diet for weight loss.

http://www.amazon.com/s/ref=nb_sb_noss?url=search-alias%3Ddigital-text&field-

keywords=dash+diet&rh=n%3A133140011%2Ck%3Adash+
diet

Another program that many people have had good
luck with is the Atkins Diet.

http://www.atkins.com/Home.aspx

The Atkins diet is focused on making protein the
major component of your food intake. By eating a high
protein diet and cutting out most of the carbs except for
vegetables the Atkins diet is supposed to turbocharge your
metabolism to help you burn fat.

One major problem with the Atkins Diet is its focus
on protein and removing as many carbohydrates as
possible. Because it doesn't have much flexibility and
requires people to cut many of their favorite foods it is
unlikely people will stick with it over the long haul.

Terry's Story

Terry always had a problem with his weight. He was fifty years old, 5 foot, seven inches tall, and weighed 375 pounds.

For the past twenty years Terry had been telling himself he was going to lose weight. He just never got around to it. Every six months he started a new diet. Good intentions seemed to fizzle out within the first week and he was back on the same roller coaster of fast food and junk foods.

Six months ago he was startled or maybe shamed is a better word into taking a good look at himself.

Terry was at the grocery store and he overheard a mother shushing her two young daughters. They were pointing at him and he heard something about the "fat boy" they saw.

Terry took it pretty hard. He'd always been self-conscious about his size and what the two girls said really gnawed at him. He sat up most of the night thinking about it.

The next morning he made up his mind he "wasn't going to be that guy anymore."

"I made an appointment with my doctor that day," said Terry, "and I told him, 'I can't live like this anymore.'" I was hoping they could cut the fat out or suck it out with liposuction. Whatever it took I was ready for it. I told him I wanted my stomach stapled.

"My doctor looked me in the eye and he said we could do that but first he wanted to know if I'd ever talked with a nutritionist, or ever really stuck to a diet and exercise plan before.

"He said it would be better for my health if I could do it without surgery. We fought about it for a good half hour or more. I finally agreed to talk with a nutritionist and get help with my eating problems. He also wanted me to start exercising; nothing strenuous at first; je just wanted me to get out of my chair and get moving. He had a trainer he wanted me to work with on that.

"The nutritionist had me write down everything I ate the week before I came in. When I got there she figured it out. I was eating 4,000 to 5,000 calories per day between all of my snacks and meals.

"She showed me the charts. I should have been eating about 2,000 to 2,200 calories per day. She didn't judge me or say I was bad, she just showed me the information and let me figure it out for myself.

"The nutritionist decided we should construct an eating plan over several visits. She told me the reason I failed on my other diets attempts was because I tried to cut out all of the foods I really liked. Her suggestion was I ease into eating less over a four to five week period. That way I wouldn't feel like I was depriving or starving myself.

"She didn't tell me I couldn't eat burgers, fries, or candy bars. She suggested I should go ahead and have them whenever I felt the urge but only take three or four bites and never ever eat more than half.

"Her advice was right on the money. That first month I had my favorite foods several times but I never had more than a few bites. It bought me time to gradually change my habits.

"By the time I got to my second month on the diet I was doing it. I was eating the right foods and never over 2,000 calories a day. Once a month I gave myself a cheat day but I stuck to having just a few bites of my favorite foods.

"My trainer was very much like the nutritionist. He told me not to rush into anything or push myself too hard. He wanted me to start moving. Most of that first month he had me park farther out in the parking lot at work and when I went out shopping at stores or the mall.

"He told me to start walking. At first I could only go five or ten minutes before I was out of breath and panting. By the end of the first week I was able to walk about fifteen minutes straight. By the end of the first month I could walk a mile in just under a half hour.

"More importantly when the nurse weighed me at the doctor's office the next month I had lost seventeen pounds.

"That was more than I ever lost in ten years on fifteen different diets."

Terry lost 62 pounds in the last six months. He has 138 pound to go to reach his target weight of 175 pounds.

The good news is this time he's confident he's going to do it. His team is behind him 100%. In fact Terry is sure that he couldn't have made it this far without his doctor, trainer, and nutritionist. They all worked together to help him reach his goal, and just as important, they encouraged him even when he fell off the wagon and overate or missed a workout.

Terry has this one piece of advice for anyone like him who is trying to lose half their body weight,

"Assemble your team, and work with them to make sure you succeed. I was lucky to get a great team on the first try. If yours isn't helping you put together a new team that will.

"And, oh yeah, hang in there. It really can happen!"

Step 6 – Get Started

Even if you weigh over 400 pounds you don't have to do the impossible to improve your situation. Aim to lose forty pounds. When you've done that adjust your sights and do it again.

Losing as little as ten percent of your body weight, can totally change your life and your health.

Over the long run a series of baby steps will help you achieve any goal you set.

Best Health Tips Ever

1) **Get a dog**.

You wouldn't believe how many people have totally transformed their lives by doing nothing other than walking their dog.

2) **Don't go on a diet**

Don't go on a diet. Continue eating your favorite foods, just eat less of them.

3) **Resolve to add a good habit**, instead of deciding to give up your bad habits.

Don't force yourself to give up that candy bar you eat every day. Decide you're going to eat an apple or orange every day for a snack and eventually you will find yourself getting healthier despite the candy bar.

4) **Don't go it alone**.

Assemble your own fitness team. Include your doctor, a nutritionist, and a trainer. They can help you over the speed bumps you're bound to encounter in your journey towards a fitter you.

5) **Don't let minor setbacks derail your progress**.

It's normal to go off on a binge for a weekend or to stop walking or working out for several days or a week. The thing to tell yourself is that it's ok, then pick yourself up and get started again.

6) **Get started today!**

This is the one that keeps most guys from getting fit. Don't tell yourself you will start tomorrow, or next week, or next month.

There's no better time than today to get started with your fitness plan.

Thank you for purchasing this book. **Fuck Fat! How Everyday Guy's Over 50 are Losing Weight & Changing Their Lives** is an attempt to bring you easy to implement solutions for improving your health.

 While no book can guarantee you success, the author and publisher have made every attempt to bring you the latest information that has been found to work for other men who are striving to stay fit after age 50. As with anything else in life results can vary, based on the time you invest and your approach to implementing the various ideas and strategies given.

If you find the contents helpful, please consider taking a few moments to leave a review.

Your comments will help other readers decide if this book may be useful to them in their job search. They will also help me to catch errors or omissions in this book, and to correct them as quickly as possible.

If you really like what you read, and are feeling a little extra love, help me get the message out there. Tweet and share this book with all of your friends on Facebook. If you know someone approaching 50 who could use a little help losing weight gift them a copy or two.

If you have any comments or questions, feel free to contact me at nick@digitalhistoryproject.com. Any corrections will be addressed in future editions.

Before starting any exercise or fitness program you should consult a doctor.